Step-by-S
Vegan Recipes

Lose Weight Quickly with a

Step-by-Step Vegan Recipes Guide.

Cruelty-free Dishes with Wholefood

Proteins, Low-Carb High-fat Combo

Franck Renner

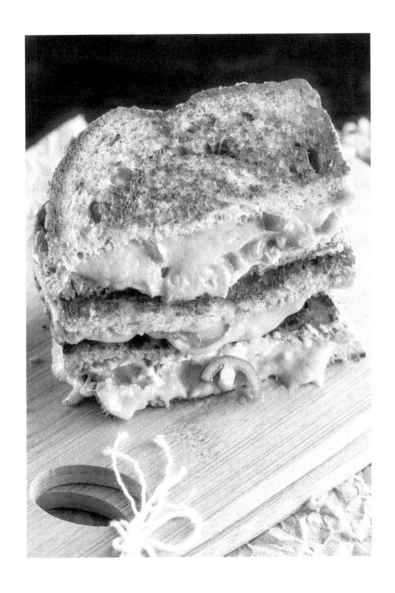

Table of Contents

CONCLUSION 114

copy and is only allowed with the express written consent from the Publisher. All additional right reserved.

The information in the following pages is broadly considered a truthful and accurate account of facts and as such, any inattention, use, or misuse of the information in question by the reader will render any resulting actions solely under their purview. There are no scenarios in which the publisher or the original author of this work can be in any fashion deemed liable for any hardship or damages that may befall them after undertaking information described herein.

Additionally, the information in the following pages is intended only for informational purposes and should thus be thought of as universal. As befitting its nature, it is presented without assurance regarding its prolonged validity or interim quality. Trademarks that are mentioned are done without written consent and can in no way be considered an endorsement from the trademark holder.

—

INTRODUCTION

The Merriam Webster Dictionary defines a vegetarian as one contains a wholly of vegetables, grains, nuts, fruits, and sometimes eggs or dairy products. It has also been described as a plant-based diet that relies wholly on plant-foods such as fruits, whole grains, herbs, vegetables, nuts, seeds, and spices. Whatever way you want to look at it, the reliance wholly on plants stands the vegetarian diet out from other types of diets. People become vegetarians for different reasons. Some take up this nutritional plan for medical or health reasons. For example, people suffering from cardiovascular diseases or who stand the risk of developing such diseases are usually advised to refrain from meat generally and focus on a plant-based diet, rich in fruits and vegetables. Some other individuals become vegetarians for religious or ethical reasons.

On this side of the spectrum are Hinduism, Jainism, Buddhism, Seventh-Day Adventists, and some other religions. It is believed that being a vegetarian is part of being holy and keeping with the ideals of non-violence. For ethical reasons, some animal rights activists are also vegetarians based on the belief that animals have rights and should not be slaughtered for food. Yet another set of persons become vegetarians based on food preference. Such individuals are naturally more disposed to a plant-based diet and find meat and other related food products less pleasurable. Some refrain from meat as a protest against climate change. This is based on the environmental concern that rearing livestock contributes to climate change and greenhouse gas emissions and the waste of natural resources in maintaining such livestock. People are usually very quick to throw words around without exactly knowing what a Vegetarian Diet means. In the same vein, the term "vegetarian" has become a popular one in recent years. What exactly does this word connote, and what does it not mean?

At its simplest, the word "vegetarian" refers to a person who refrains from eating meat, beef, pork, lard, chicken, or even fish. Depending on the kind of vegetarian it is, however, a vegetarian could either eat or exclude from his diet animal products. Animal products would refer to foods such as eggs, dairy products, and even honey! A vegetarian diet would, therefore, refer to the nutritional plan of the void of meat. It is the eating lifestyle of individuals who depend on plant-based foods for nutrition. It excludes animal products, particularly meat - a common denominator for all kinds of Vegetarians - from their diets. A vegetarian could also be defined as a meal plan that consists of foods coming majorly from plants to the exclusion of meat, poultry, and seafood.

This kind of Vegetarian diet usually contains no animal protein.

It is completely understandable from the discussion so far that the term "vegetarian" is more or less a blanket term covering different plant-based diets. While reliance majorly on plant foods is consistent in all the different types of vegetarians, they have some underlying differences. The different types of vegetarians are discussed below:

Veganism: This is undoubtedly the strictest type of vegetarian diet. Vegans exclude the any animal product. It goes as far as avoiding animal-derived ingredients contained in processed foods. Whether its meat, poultry products like eggs, dairy products inclusive of milk, honey, or even gelatin, they all are excluded from the vegans.

Some vegans go beyond nutrition and go as far as refusing to wear clothes that contain animal products. This means such vegans do not wear leather, wool, or silk.

Lacto-vegetarian: This kind of vegetarian excludes meat, fish, and poultry. However, it allows the inclusion of dairy products such as milk, yogurt, cheese, and butter. The hint is perhaps in the name since Lacto means milk in Latin.

Ovo-Vegetarian: Meat and dairy products are excluded under this diet, but eggs could be consumed. Ovo means egg.

Lacto-Ovo Vegetarian: This appears to be the hybrid of the Ovo Vegetarian and the Lacto-Vegetarian. This is the most famous type of vegetarian diet and is usually what comes to mind when people think of the Vegetarian. This type of Vegetarian bars all kinds of meat but allows for the consumption of eggs and dairy products.

Pollotarian: This vegetarian allows the consumption of chicken.

Pescatarian: This refers to the vegetarian that consumes fish. More people are beginning to subscribe to this kind of diet due to health reasons.

Flexitarian: Flexitarians are individuals who prefer plant-based foods to meat but have no problem eating meats once in a while. They are also referred to as semi-vegetarians.

Raw Vegan: This is also called the raw food and consists of a vegan that is yet to be processed and has also not been heated over 46 C. This kind of diet has its root in the belief that nutrients and minerals present in the plant diet are lost when cooked on temperature above 46 C and could also become harmful to the body.

Moroccan Vermicelli Vegetable Soup

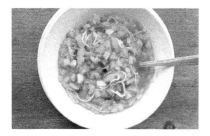

Preparation Time: 5 minutes

Cooking Time: 35 minutes

Servings: 4 to 6

Ingredients:

- 1 tablespoon olive oil
- 1 small onion, chopped
- 1 large carrot, chopped
- 1 celery rib, chopped
- 3 small zucchini, cut into 1/4-inch dice
- 1 (28-ounce) can diced tomatoes, drained
- 2 tablespoons tomato paste
- 11/2 cups cooked or 1 (15.5-ounce) can chickpeas, drained and rinsed
- 2 teaspoons smoked paprika
- 1 teaspoon ground cumin
- 1 teaspoon za'atar spice (optional)
- 1/4 teaspoon ground cayenne

- 6 cups vegetable broth, homemade (see light vegetable broth) or store-bought, or water

- Salt

- 4 ounces vermicelli

- 2 tablespoons minced fresh cilantro, for garnish

Directions:

1. In a large soup pot, heat the oil over medium heat. Add the onion, carrot, and celery. Cover and cook until softened, about 5 minutes. Stir in the zucchini, tomatoes, tomato paste, chickpeas, paprika, cumin, za'atar, and cayenne.

2. Add the broth and salt to taste. Bring to a boil, then reduce heat to low and simmer, uncovered, until the vegetables are tender, about 30 minutes.

3. Shortly before serving, stir in the vermicelli and cook until the noodles are tender, about 5 minutes. Ladle the soup into bowls, garnish with cilantro, and serve.

Nutrition: Calories: 236 kcal Fat: 1.8g Carbs: 48.3g Protein: 7g

Tomato Gazpacho

Preparation Time: 30 minutes

Cooking Time: 55 minutes

Servings: 6

Ingredients:

- 2 Tablespoons + 1 Teaspoon Red Wine Vinegar, Divided
- ½ Teaspoon Pepper
- 1 Teaspoon Sea Salt
- 1 Avocado,
- ¼ Cup Basil, Fresh & Chopped
- 3 Tablespoons + 2 Teaspoons Olive Oil, Divided
- 1 Clove Garlic, crushed
- 1 Red Bell Pepper, Sliced & Seeded
- 1 Cucumber, Chunked
- 2 ½ lbs. Large Tomatoes, Cored & Chopped

Directions:

1. Place half of your cucumber, bell pepper, and ¼ cup of each tomato in a bowl, covering. Set it in the fried.

2. Puree your remaining tomatoes, cucumber and bell pepper with garlic, three tablespoons oil, two tablespoons of vinegar, sea salt and black pepper into a blender, blending until smooth. Transfer it to a bowl, and chill for two hours.

3. Chop the avocado, adding it to your chopped vegetables, adding your remaining oil, vinegar, salt, pepper and basil.

4. Ladle your tomato puree mixture into bowls, and serve with chopped vegetables as a salad.

5. Interesting Facts:

6. Avocados themselves are ranked within the top five of the healthiest foods on the planet, so you know that the oil that is produced from them is too. It is loaded with healthy fats and essential fatty acids. Like race bran oil it is perfect to cook with as well! Bonus: Helps in the prevention of diabetes and lowers cholesterol levels.

Nutrition: Calories 201 Protein 23g Fat 4 Carbs 2

Tomato Pumpkin Soup

Preparation Time: 25 minutes

Cooking Time: 25 minutes

Servings: 4

Ingredients:

- 2 cups pumpkin, diced
- 1/2 cup tomato, chopped
- 1/2 cup onion, chopped
- 1 1/2 tsp curry powder
- 1/2 tsp paprika
- 2 cups vegetable stock
- 1 tsp olive oil
- 1/2 tsp garlic, minced

Directions:

1. In a saucepan, add oil, garlic, and onion and sauté for 3 minutes over medium heat.
2. Add remaining ingredients into the saucepan and bring to boil.
3. Reduce heat and cover and simmer for 10 minutes.
4. Puree the soup using a blender until smooth.
5. Stir well and serve warm.

Nutrition: Calories: 340 Protein: 50 g Carbohydrate: 14 g Fat: 10g

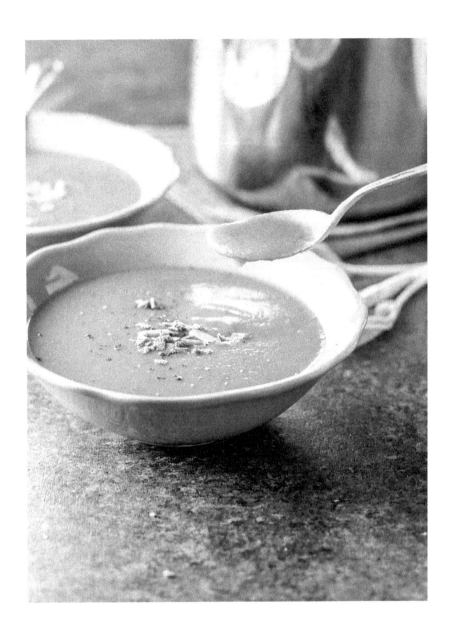

Creamy Garlic Onion Soup

Preparation Time: 45 minutes

Cooking Time: 25 minutes

Servings: 4

Ingredients:

- 1 onion, sliced
- 4 cups vegetable stock
- 1 1/2 tbsp. olive oil
- 1 shallot, sliced
- 2 garlic clove, chopped
- 1 leek, sliced
- Salt

Directions:

1. Add stock and olive oil in a saucepan and bring to boil.
2. Add remaining ingredients and stir well.
3. Cover and simmer for 25 minutes.
4. Puree the soup using an immersion blender until smooth.
5. Stir well and serve warm.

Nutrition: Calories 115 Protein 30g Fat 0 Carbs 3

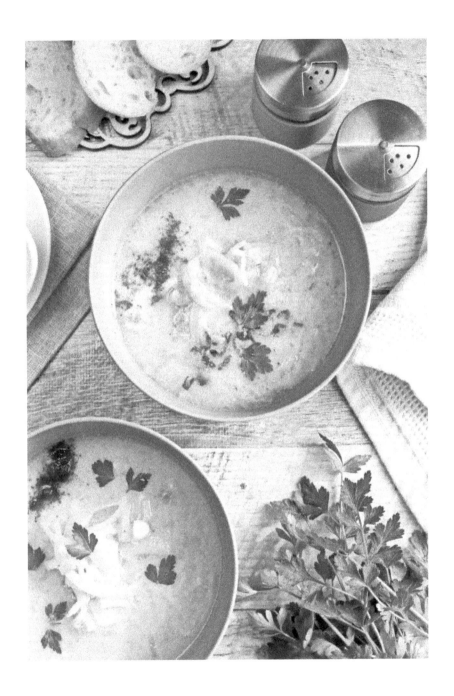

Avocado Broccoli Soup

Preparation Time: 20 minutes

Cooking Time: 5 minutes

Servings: 4

Ingredients:

- 2 cups broccoli florets, chopped
- 5 cups vegetable broth
- 2 avocados, chopped
- Pepper
- Salt

Directions:

1. Cook broccoli in boiling water for 5 minutes. Drain well.
2. Add broccoli, vegetable broth, avocados, pepper, and salt to the blender and blend until smooth.
3. Stir well and serve warm.

Nutrition: Calories 265 Protein 35g Fat 13 Carbs 5

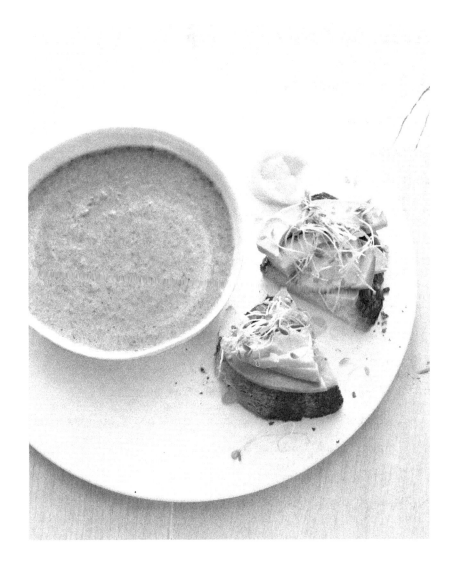

Green Spinach Kale Soup

Preparation Time: 10 minutes

Cooking Time: 5 minutes

Servings: 6

Ingredients:

- 2 avocados
- 8 oz. spinach
- 8 oz. kale
- 1 fresh lime juice
- 1 cup water
- 3 1/3 cup coconut milk
- 3 oz. olive oil
- 1/4 tsp pepper
- 1 tsp salt

Directions:

1. Heat olive oil in a saucepan over medium heat.
2. Add kale and spinach to the saucepan and sauté for 2-3 minutes. Remove saucepan from heat. Add coconut milk, spices, avocado, and water. Stir well.
3. Puree the soup using an immersion blender until smooth and creamy. Add fresh lime juice and stir well.
4. Serve and enjoy.

Nutrition: Calories: 312 Protein: 9g Fat: 10 Carbs: 22

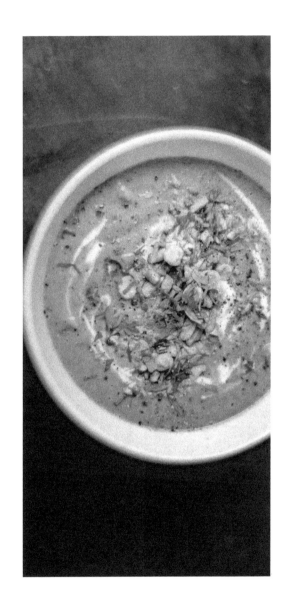

Cauliflower Asparagus Soup

Preparation Time: 10 minutes

Cooking Time: 30 minutes

Servings: 4

Ingredients:

- 20 asparagus spears, chopped
- 4 cups vegetable stock
- ½ cauliflower head, chopped
- 2 garlic cloves, chopped
- 1 tbsp. coconut oil
- Pepper
- Salt

Directions:

1. Heat coconut oil in a large saucepan over medium heat.
2. Add garlic and sauté until softened.
3. Add cauliflower, vegetable stock, pepper, and salt. Stir well and bring to boil.
4. Reduce heat to low and simmer for 20 minutes.
5. Add chopped asparagus and cook until softened.
6. Puree the soup using an immersion blender until smooth and creamy.
7. Stir well and serve warm.

Nutrition: Kcal: 298 Carbohydrates: 26 g Protein: 21 g Fat:9 g

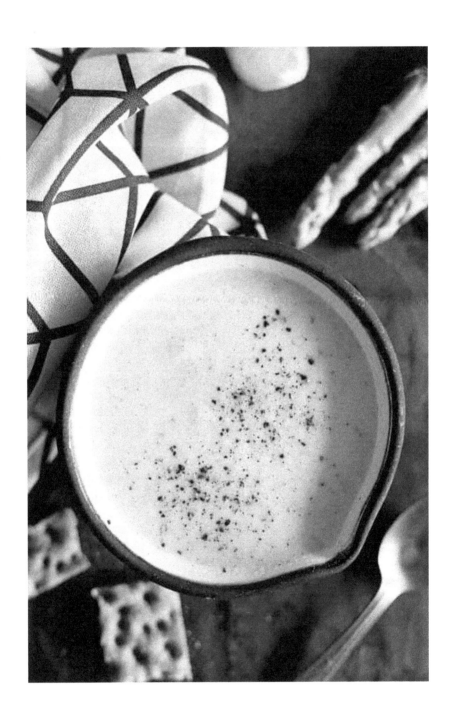

African Pineapple Peanut Stew

Preparation Time: 10 minutes

Cooking Time: 20 minutes

Servings: 4

Ingredients:

- 4 cups sliced kale
- 1 cup chopped onion
- 1/2 cup peanut butter
- 1 tbsp. hot pepper sauce or 1 tbsp. Tabasco sauce
- 2 minced garlic cloves
- 1/2 cup chopped cilantro
- 2 cups pineapple, undrained, canned & crushed
- 1 tbsp. vegetable oil

Directions:

1. In a saucepan (preferably covered), sauté the garlic and onions in the oil until the onions are lightly browned, approximately 10 minutes, stirring often.

2. Wash the kale, till the time the onions are sauté.

3. Get rid of the stems. Mound the leaves on a cutting surface & slice crosswise into slices (preferably 1" thick).

4. Now put the pineapple and juice to the onions & bring to a simmer. Stir the kale in, cover and simmer until just tender, stirring frequently, approximately 5 minutes.

5. Mix in the hot pepper sauce, peanut butter & simmer for more 5 minutes.

6. Add salt according to your taste.

Nutrition: Kcal: 402 Carbohydrates: 7 g Protein: 21 g Fat: 34 g

Cabbage & Beet Stew

Preparation Time: 20 minutes

Cooking Time: 10 minutes

Servings: 4

Ingredients:

- 2 Tablespoons Olive Oil
- 3 Cups Vegetable Broth
- 2 Tablespoons Lemon Juice, Fresh
- ½ Teaspoon Garlic Powder
- ½ Cup Carrots, Shredded
- 2 Cups Cabbage, Shredded
- 1 Cup Beets, Shredded
- Dill for Garnish
- ½ Teaspoon Onion Powder
- Sea Salt & Black Pepper to Taste

Directions:

1. Heat oil in a pot, and then sauté your vegetables.
2. Pour your broth in, mixing in your seasoning. Simmer until it's cooked through, and then top with dill.

Nutrition: Kcal: 263 Carbohydrates: 8 g Protein: 20.3 g Fat: 24 g

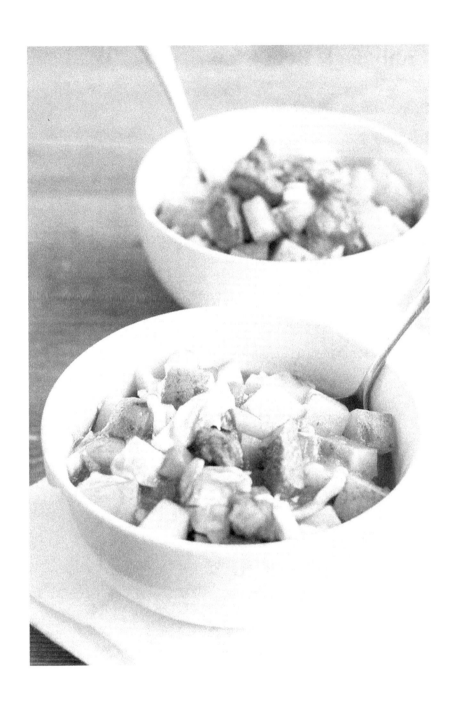

Basil Tomato Soup

Preparation Time: 10 minutes

Cooking Time: 10 minutes

Servings: 6

Ingredients:

- 28 oz. can tomatoes
- ¼ cup basil pesto
- ¼ tsp dried basil leaves
- 1 tsp apple cider vinegar
- 2 tbsp. erythritol
- ¼ tsp garlic powder
- ½ tsp onion powder
- 2 cups water
- 1 ½ tsp kosher salt

Directions:

1. Add tomatoes, garlic powder, onion powder, water, and salt in a saucepan.
2. Bring to boil over medium heat. Reduce heat and simmer for 2 minutes.
3. Remove saucepan from heat and puree the soup using a blender until smooth.
4. Stir in pesto, dried basil, vinegar, and erythritol.
5. Stir well and serve warm.

Nutrition: Kcal: 662 Carbohydrates: 18 g Protein: 8 g Fat: 55 g

Mushroom & Broccoli Soup

Preparation Time: 20 minutes

Cooking Time: 45 minutes

Servings: 8

Ingredients:

- 1 bundle broccoli (around 1-1/2 pounds)
- 1 tablespoon canola oil
- 1/2 pound cut crisp mushrooms
- 1 tablespoon diminished sodium soy sauce
- 2 medium carrots, finely slashed
- 2 celery ribs, finely slashed
- 1/4 cup finely slashed onion
- 1 garlic clove, minced
- 1 container (32 ounces) vegetable juices
- 2 cups of water
- 2 tablespoons lemon juice

Directions:

1. Cut broccoli florets into reduced down pieces. Strip and hack stalks.

2. In an enormous pot, heat oil over medium-high warmth; saute mushrooms until delicate, 4-6 minutes. Mix in soy sauce; expel from skillet.

3. In the same container, join broccoli stalks, carrots, celery, onion, garlic, soup, and water; heat to the point of boiling. Diminish heat; stew, revealed, until vegetables are relaxed, 25-30 minutes.

4. Puree soup utilizing a drenching blender. Or then again, cool marginally and puree the soup in a blender; come back to the dish.

5. Mix in florets and mushrooms; heat to the point of boiling. Lessen warmth to medium; cook until broccoli is delicate, 8-10 minutes, blending infrequently. Mix in lemon juice.

Nutrition: Kcal: 830 Carbohydrates: 8 g Protein: 45 g Fat: 64 g

Creamy Cauliflower Pakora Soup

Preparation Time: 20 minutes

Cooking Time: 20 minutes

Servings: 8

Ingredients:

- 1 huge head cauliflower, cut into little florets
- 5 medium potatoes, stripped and diced
- 1 huge onion, diced
- 4 medium carrots, stripped and diced
- 2 celery ribs, diced
- 1 container (32 ounces) vegetable stock
- 1 teaspoon garam masala
- 1 teaspoon garlic powder
- 1 teaspoon ground coriander
- 1 teaspoon ground turmeric
- 1 teaspoon ground cumin
- 1 teaspoon pepper
- 1 teaspoon salt
- 1/2 teaspoon squashed red pepper chips
- Water or extra vegetable stock
- New cilantro leaves
- Lime wedges, discretionary

Directions:

1. In a Dutch stove over medium-high warmth, heat initial 14 fixings to the point of boiling. Cook and mix until vegetables are delicate, around 20 minutes. Expel from heat; cool marginally. Procedure in groups in a blender or nourishment processor until smooth. Modify consistency as wanted with water (or extra stock). Sprinkle with new cilantro. Serve hot, with lime wedges whenever wanted.

2. Stop alternative: Before including cilantro, solidify cooled soup in cooler compartments. To utilize, in part defrost in cooler medium-term.

3. Warmth through in a pan, blending every so often and including a little water if fundamental. Sprinkle with cilantro. Whenever wanted, present with lime wedges.

Nutrition: Kcal: 248 Carbohydrates: 7 g Protein: 1 g Fat: 19 g

Garden Vegetable and Herb Soup

Preparation Time: 20 minutes

Cooking Time: 30 minutes

Servings: 8

Ingredients:

- 2 tablespoons olive oil

- 2 medium onions, hacked

- 2 huge carrots, cut

- 1 pound red potatoes (around 3 medium), cubed

- 2 cups of water

- 1 can (14-1/2 ounces) diced tomatoes in sauce

- 1-1/2 cups vegetable soup

- 1-1/2 teaspoons garlic powder

- 1 teaspoon dried basil

- 1/2 teaspoon salt

- 1/2 teaspoon paprika

- 1/4 teaspoon dill weed

- 1/4 teaspoon pepper

- 1 medium yellow summer squash, split and cut

- 1 medium zucchini, split and cut

Directions:

1. In a huge pan, heat oil over medium warmth. Include onions and carrots; cook and mix until onions are delicate, 4-6 minutes. Include potatoes and cook 2 minutes. Mix in water, tomatoes, juices, and seasonings.
2. Heat to the point of boiling. Diminish heat; stew, revealed, until potatoes and carrots are delicate, 9 minutes.
3. Include yellow squash and zucchini; cook until vegetables are delicate, 9 minutes longer. Serve or, whenever wanted, puree blend in clusters, including extra stock until desired consistency is accomplished.

Nutrition: Kcal: 252 Carbohydrates: 12 g Protein: 1 g Fat: 11 g

The Mediterranean Delight with Fresh Vinaigrette

Preparation Time: 5 minutes

Cooking Time: 10 minutes

Servings: 2

Ingredients:

- Herbed citrus vinaigrette:
- 1 tablespoon of lemon juice
- 2 tablespoons of orange juice
- ½ teaspoon of lemon zest
- ½ teaspoon of orange zest
- 2 tablespoons of olive oil
- 1 tablespoon of finely chopped fresh oregano leaves
- Salt to taste
- Black pepper to taste
- 2-3 tablespoons of freshly julienned mint leaves
- Salad:
- 1 freshly diced medium-sized cucumber
- 2 cups of cooked and rinsed chickpeas
- ½ cup of freshly diced red onion
- 2 freshly diced medium-sized tomatoes
- 1 freshly diced red bell pepper

- ¼ cup of green olives
- ½ cup of pomegranates

Directions:

1. In a large salad bowl, add the juice and zest of both the lemon and the orange along with oregano and olive oil. Whisk together so that they are mixed well. Season the vinaigrette with salt and pepper to taste.

2. After draining the chickpeas, add them to the dressing. Then, add the onions. Give them a thorough mix, so that the onion and chickpeas absorb the flavors.

3. Now, chop the rest of the veggies and start adding them to the salad bowl. Give them a good toss.

4. Lastly, add the olives and fresh mint. Adjust the salt and pepper as required.

5. Serve this Mediterranean delight chilled — a cool summer salad that is good for the tummy and the soul.

Nutrition: Kcal: 286 Carbohydrates: 29 g Protein: 1 g Fat: 11 g

Moroccan Vegetable Stew

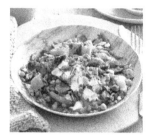

Preparation Time: 5 minutes

Cooking Time: 35 minutes

Servings: 4

Ingredients:

- 1 tablespoon olive oil

- 2 medium yellow onions, chopped

- 2 medium carrots, cut into 1/2-inch dice

- 1/2 teaspoon ground cumin

- 1/2 teaspoon ground cinnamon or allspice

- 1/2 teaspoon ground ginger

- 1/2 teaspoon sweet or smoked paprika

- 1/2 teaspoon saffron or turmeric

- 1 (14.5-ounce) can diced tomatoes, undrained

- 8 ounces green beans, trimmed and cut into 1-inch pieces

- 2 cups peeled, seeded, and diced winter squash

- 1 large russet or other baking potato, peeled and cut into 1/2-inch dice

- 11/2 cups vegetable broth
- 11/2 cups cooked or 1 (15.5-ounce) can chickpeas, drained and rinsed
- ¾ cup frozen peas
- 1/2 cup pitted dried plums (prunes)
- 1 teaspoon lemon zest
- Salt and freshly ground black pepper
- 1/2 cup pitted green olives
- 1 tablespoon minced fresh cilantro or parsley, for garnish
- 1/2 cup toasted slivered almonds, for garnish

Directions:

1. In a large saucepan, heat the oil over medium heat. Add the onions and carrots, cover, and cook for 5 minutes. Stir in the cumin, cinnamon, ginger, paprika, and saffron. Cook, uncovered, stirring, for 30 seconds.

2. Add the tomatoes, green beans, squash, potato, and broth and bring to a boil. Reduce heat to low, cover, and simmer until the vegetables are tender, about 20 minutes.

3. Add the chickpeas, peas, dried plums, and lemon zest. Season with salt and pepper to taste. Stir in the olives and simmer, uncovered, until the flavors are blended, about 10 minutes. Sprinkle with cilantro and almonds and serve immediately.

Nutrition: Calories: 71 kcal Fat: 2.8g Carbs: 9.8g Protein: 3.7g

Basic Recipe for Vegetable Broth

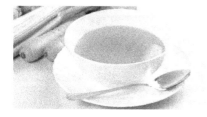

Preparation Time: 10 Minutes

Cooking Time: 60 Minutes

Servings: Makes 2 Quarts

Ingredients:

- 8 cups Water

- 1 Onion, chopped

- 4 Garlic cloves, crushed

- 2 Celery Stalks, chopped

- Pinch of Salt

- 1 Carrot, chopped

- Dash of Pepper

- 1 Potato, medium & chopped

- 1 tbsp. Soy Sauce

- 3 Bay Leaves

Directions:

1. To make the vegetable broth, you need to place all of the ingredients in a deep saucepan.

2. Heat the pan over a medium-high heat. Bring the vegetable mixture to a boil.

3. Once it starts boiling, lower the heat to medium-low and allow it to simmer for at least an hour or so. Cover it with a lid.

4. When the time is up, pass it through a filter and strain the vegetables, garlic, and bay leaves.

5. Allow the stock to cool completely and store in an air-tight container.

Nutrition: Calories: 44 kcal Fat: 0.6g Carbs: 9.7g Protein: 0.9g

Cucumber Dill Gazpacho

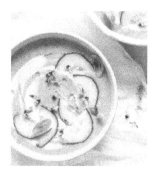

Preparation Time: 10 Minutes

Cooking Time: 2 hours

Serving Size: 4

Ingredients:

- 4 large cucumbers, peeled, deseeded, and chopped
- 1/8 tsp salt
- 1 tsp chopped fresh dill + more for garnishing
- 2 tbsp. freshly squeezed lemon juice
- 1 ½ cups green grape, seeds removed
- 3 tbsp. extra virgin olive oil
- 1 garlic clove, minced

Directions:

1. Add all the ingredients to a food processor and blend until smooth.
2. Pour the soup into serving bowls and chill for 1 to 2 hours.
3. Garnish with dill and serve chilled.

Nutrition: Calories: 236 kcal Fat: 1.8g Carbs: 48.3g Protein: 7g

Red Lentil Soup

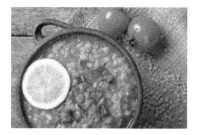

Preparation Time: 5 Minutes

Cooking Time: 25 Minutes

Servings: Makes 6 cups

Ingredients:

- 2 tbsp. Nutritional Yeast
- 1 cup Red Lentil, washed
- ½ tbsp. Garlic, minced
- 4 cups Vegetable Stock
- 1 tsp. Salt
- 2 cups Kale, shredded
- 3 cups Mixed Vegetables

Directions:

1. To start with, place all ingredients needed to make the soup in a large pot.
2. Heat the pot over medium-high heat and bring the mixture to a boil.

3. Once it starts boiling, lower the heat to low. Allow the soup to simmer.

4. Simmer it for 1o to 15 minutes or until cooked.

5. Serve and enjoy.

Nutrition: Calories: 212 kcal Fat: 11.9g Carbs: 31.7g Protein: 7.3g

Spinach and Kale Soup

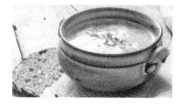

Preparation Time: 5 Minutes

Cooking Time: 5 Minutes

Servings: 2

Ingredients:

- 3 oz. vegan butter
- 1 cup fresh spinach, chopped coarsely
- 1 cup fresh kale, chopped coarsely
- 1 large avocado
- 3 tbsp. chopped fresh mint leaves
- 3 ½ cups coconut cream
- 1 cup vegetable broth
- Salt and black pepper to taste
- 1 lime, juiced

Directions:

1. Melt the vegan butter in a medium pot over medium heat and sauté the kale and spinach until wilted, 3 minutes. Turn the heat off.

2. Stir in the remaining ingredients and using an immersion blender, puree the soup until smooth.

3. Dish the soup and serve warm.

Nutrition: Calories 380 Fat 10 g Protein 20 g Carbohydrates 30 g

Coconut and Grilled Vegetable Soup

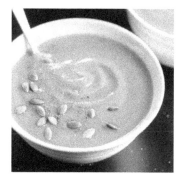

Preparation Time: 10 Minutes

Cooking Time: 45 Minutes

Servings: 4

Ingredients:

- 2 small red onions cut into wedges
- 2 garlic cloves
- 10 oz. butternut squash, peeled and chopped
- 10 oz. pumpkins, peeled and chopped
- 4 tbsp. melted vegan butter
- Salt and black pepper to taste
- 1 cup of water
- 1 cup unsweetened coconut milk
- 1 lime juiced
- ¾ cup vegan mayonnaise
- Toasted pumpkin seeds for garnishing

Directions:

1. Preheat the oven to 400 F.

2. On a baking sheet, spread the onions, garlic, butternut squash, and pumpkins and drizzle half of the butter on top. Season with salt, black pepper, and rub the seasoning well onto the vegetables. Roast in the oven for 45 minutes or until the vegetables are golden brown and softened.

3. Transfer the vegetables to a pot; add the remaining ingredients except for the pumpkin seeds and using an immersion blender puree the ingredients until smooth.

4. Dish the soup, garnish with the pumpkin seeds and serve warm.

Nutrition: Calories 290 Fat 10 g Protein 30 g Carbohydrates 0 g

Broccoli Fennel Soup

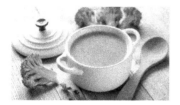

Preparation Time: 15 Minutes

Cooking Time: 10 Minutes

Servings: 4

Ingredients:

- 1 fennel bulb, white and green parts coarsely chopped
- 10 oz. broccoli, cut into florets
- 3 cups vegetable stock
- Salt and freshly ground black pepper
- 1 garlic clove
- 1 cup dairy-free cream cheese
- 3 oz. vegan butter
- ½ cup chopped fresh oregano

Directions:

1. In a medium pot, combine the fennel, broccoli, vegetable stock, salt, and black pepper. Bring to a boil until the vegetables soften, 10 to 15 minutes.

2. Stir in the remaining ingredients and simmer the soup for 3 to 5 minutes.

3. Adjust the taste with salt and black pepper, and dish the soup.

4. Serve warm.

Nutrition: Calories 240 Fat 0 g Protein 0 g Carbohydrates 20 g

Tofu Goulash Soup

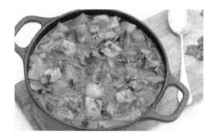

Preparation Time: 35 Minutes

Cooking Time: 20 Minutes

Servings: 4

Ingredients:

- 4¼ oz. vegan butter
- 1 white onion, chopped
- 2 garlic cloves, minced
- 1 ½ cups butternut squash
- 1 red bell pepper, deseeded and chopped
- 1 tbsp. paprika powder
- ¼ tsp red chili flakes
- 1 tbsp. dried basil
- ½ tbsp. crushed cardamom seeds
- Salt and black pepper to taste

- 1 ½ cups crushed tomatoes
- 3 cups vegetable broth
- 1½ tsp red wine vinegar
- Chopped parsley to serve

Directions:

1. Place the tofu between two paper towels and allow draining of water for 30 minutes. After, crumble the tofu and set aside.
2. Melt the vegan butter in a large pot over medium heat and sauté the onion and garlic until the veggies are fragrant and soft, 3 minutes.
3. Stir in the tofu and cook until golden brown, 3 minutes.
4. Add the butternut squash, bell pepper, paprika, red chili flakes, basil, cardamom seeds, salt, and black pepper. Cook for 2 minutes to release some flavor and mix in the tomatoes and 2 cups of vegetable broth.
5. Close the lid, bring the soup to a boil, and then simmer for 10 minutes.
6. Stir in the remaining vegetable broth, the red wine vinegar, and adjust the taste with salt and black pepper.
7. Dish the soup, garnish with the parsley and serve warm.

Nutrition: Calories 320 Fat 10 g Protein 10 g Carbohydrates 20 g

Pesto Pea Soup

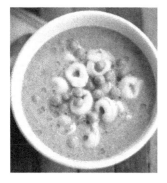

Preparation Time: 10 Minutes

Cooking Time: 20 Minutes

Servings: 4

Ingredients:

- 2 cups Water

- 8 oz. Tortellini

- ¼ cup Pesto

- 1 Onion, small & finely chopped

- 1 lb. Peas, frozen

- 1 Carrot, medium & finely chopped

- 1 ¾ cup Vegetable Broth, less sodium

- 1 Celery Rib, medium & finely chopped

Directions:

1. To start with, boil the water in a large pot over a medium-high heat.

2. Next, stir in the tortellini to the pot and cook it following the instructions given in the packet.

3. In the meantime, cook the onion, celery, and carrot in a deep saucepan along with the water and broth.

4. Cook the celery-onion mixture for 6 minutes or until softened.

5. Now, spoon in the peas and allow it to simmer while keeping it uncovered.

6. Cook the peas for few minutes or until they are bright green and soft.

7. Then, spoon in the pesto to the peas mixture. Combine well.

8. Pour the mixture into a high-speed blender and blend for 2 to 3 minutes or until you get a rich, smooth soup.

9. Return the soup to the pan. Spoon in the cooked tortellini.

10. Finally, pour into a serving bowl and top with more cooked peas if desired.

11. Tip: If desired, you can season it with Maldon salt at the end.

Nutrition: Calories 100 Fat 0 g Protein 0 g Carbohydrates 0 g

Tofu and Mushroom Soup

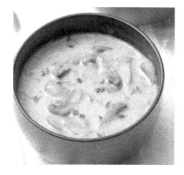

Preparation Time: 15 Minutes

Cooking Time: 10 Minutes

Servings: 4

Ingredients:

- 2 tbsp. olive oil

- 1 garlic clove, minced

- 1 large yellow onion, finely chopped

- 1 tsp freshly grated ginger

- 1 cup vegetable stock

- 2 small potatoes, peeled and chopped

- ¼ tsp salt

- ¼ tsp black pepper

- 2 (14 oz.) silken tofu, drained and rinsed

- 2/3 cup baby Bella mushrooms, sliced

- 1 tbsp. chopped fresh oregano

- 2 tbsp. chopped fresh parsley to garnish

Directions:

1. Heat the olive oil in a medium pot over medium heat and sauté the garlic, onion, and ginger until soft and fragrant.

2. Pour in the vegetable stock, potatoes, salt, and black pepper. Cook until the potatoes soften, 12 minutes.

3. Stir in the tofu and using an immersion blender, puree the ingredients until smooth.

4. Mix in the mushrooms and simmer with the pot covered until the mushrooms warm up while occasionally stirring to ensure that the tofu doesn't curdle, 7 minutes.

5. Stir oregano, and dish the soup.

6. Garnish with the parsley and serve warm.

Nutrition: Calories 310 Fat 10 g Protein 40.0 g Carbohydrates 0 g

Avocado Green Soup

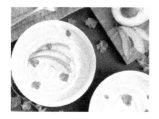

Preparation Time: 5 Minutes

Cooking Time: 5 Minutes

Servings: 4

Ingredients:

- 2 tbsp. olive oil
- 1 ½ cup fresh kale, chopped coarsely
- 1 ½ cup fresh spinach, chopped coarsely
- 3 large avocados, halved, pitted and pulp extracted
- 2 cups of soy milk
- 2 cups no-sodium vegetable broth
- 3 tbsp. chopped fresh mint leaves
- ¼ tsp salt
- ¼ tsp black pepper
- 2 limes, juiced

Directions:

1. Heat the olive oil in a medium saucepan over medium heat and mix in the kale and spinach. Cook until wilted, 3 minutes and turn off the heat.
2. Add the remaining ingredients and using an immersion blender, puree the soup until smooth.
3. Dish the soup and serve immediately.

Nutrition: Calories 400 Fat 10 g Protein 20 g Carbohydrates 30 g

Black Bean Nacho Soup

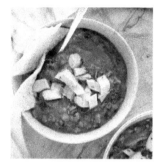

Preparation Time: 5 Minutes

Cooking Time: 30 Minutes

Servings: 4

Ingredients:

- 30 oz. Black Bean
- 1 tbsp. Olive Oil
- 2 cups Vegetable Stock
- ½ of 1 Onion, large & chopped
- 2 ½ cups Water
- 3 Garlic cloves, minced
- 14 oz. Mild Green Chillies, diced
- 1 tsp. Cumin
- 1 cup Salsa
- ½ tsp. Salt
- 16 oz. Tomato Paste
- ½ tsp. Black Pepper

Directions:

1. For making this delicious fare, heat oil in a large pot over medium-high heat.

2. Once the oil becomes hot, stir in onion and garlic to it.

3. Sauté for 4 minutes or until the onion is softened.

4. Next, spoon in chili powder, salt, cumin, and pepper to the pot. Mix well.

5. Then, stir in tomato paste, salsa, water, green chillies, and vegetable stock to onion mixture. Combine.

6. Bing the mixture to a boil. Allow the veggies to simmer.

7. When the mixture starts simmering, add the beans.

8. Bring the veggie mixture to a simmer again and lower the heat to low.

9. Finally, cook for 15 to 20 minutes and check for seasoning. Add more salt and pepper if needed.

10. Garnish with the topping of your choice. Serve it hot.

Nutrition: Calories 270 Fat 10 g Protein 10 g Carbohydrates 10 g

Potato Leek Soup

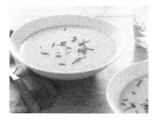

Preparation Time: 5 Minutes

Cooking Time: 5 Minutes

Servings: 4

Ingredients:

- 1 cup fresh cilantro leaves

- 6 garlic cloves, peeled

- 3 tbsp. vegetable oil

- 3 leeks, white and green parts chopped

- 2 lb. russet potatoes, peeled and chopped

- 1 tsp cumin powder

- ¼ tsp salt

- ¼ tsp black pepper

- 2 bay leaves

- 6 cups no-sodium vegetable broth

Directions:

1. In a spice blender, process the cilantro and garlic until smooth paste forms.

2. Heat the vegetable oil in a large pot and sauté the garlic mixture and leeks until the leeks are tender, 5 minutes.

3. Mix in the remaining ingredients and allow boiling until the potatoes soften, 15 minutes.

4. Turn the heat off, open the lid, remove and discard the bay leaves.

5. Using an immersion blender, puree the soup until smooth.

6. Dish the food and serve warm.

Nutrition: Calories 215 Fat 0 g Protein 10 g Carbohydrates 20.0 g

Lentil Soup

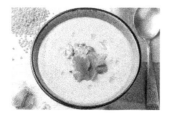

Preparation Time: 15 Minutes

Cooking Time: 25 Minutes

Servings: 4

Ingredients:

- 1 tbsp. Olive Oil
- 4 cups Vegetable Stock
- 1 Onion, finely chopped
- 2 Carrots, medium
- 1 cup Lentils, dried
- 1 tsp. Cumin

Directions:

1. To make this healthy soup, first, you need to heat the oil in a medium-sized skillet over medium heat.
2. Once the oil becomes hot, stir in the cumin and then the onions.
3. Sauté them for 3 minutes or until the onion is slightly transparent and cooked.
4. To this, add the carrots and toss them well.

5. Next, stir in the lentils. Mix well.

6. Now, pour in the vegetable stock and give a good stir until everything comes together.

7. As the soup mixture starts to boil, reduce the heat and allow it to simmer for 10 minutes while keeping the pan covered.

8. Turn off the heat and then transfer the mixture to a bowl.

9. Finally, blend it with an immersion blender or in a high-speed blender for 1 minute or until you get a rich, smooth mixture.

10. Serve it hot and enjoy.

Nutrition: Calories: 266 Fat: 13 Fiber: 8 Carbs. 10 Protein: 11

Kale White Bean Soup

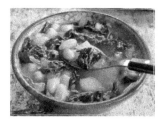

Preparation Time: 10 Minutes

Cooking Time: 45 Minutes

Servings: 4

Ingredients:

- 1 Onion, medium & finely sliced
- 3 cups Kale, coarsely chopped
- 2 tsp. Olive Oil
- 15 oz. White Beans
- 4 cups Vegetable Broth
- 4 Garlic Cloves, minced
- Sea Salt & Pepper, as needed
- 2 tsp. Rosemary, fresh & chopped
- 1 lb. White Potatoes, cubed

Directions:

1. Begin by taking a large saucepan and heat it over a medium-high heat.
2. Once the pan becomes hot, spoon in the oil.

3. Next, stir in the onion and sauté for 8 to 9 minutes or until the onions are cooked and lightly browned.

4. Then, add the garlic and rosemary to the pan.

5. Sauté for a further minute or until aromatic.

6. Now, pour in the broth along with the potatoes, black pepper, and salt. Mix well.

7. Bring the mixture to a boil, and when it starts boiling, lower the heat.

8. Allow it to simmer for 32 to 35 minutes or until the potatoes are cooked and tender.

9. After that, mash the potatoes slightly by using the back of the spoon.

10. Finally, add the kale and beans to the soup and cook for 8 minutes or until the kale is wilted.

11. Check the seasoning. Add more salt and pepper if needed.

12. Serve hot.

Nutrition: Calories: 198 Fat: 11 Fiber: 1 Carbs: 12 Protein: 12

Black Bean Mushroom Soup

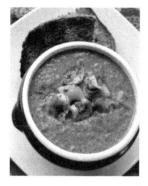

Preparation Time: 10 Minutes

Cooking Time: 40 Minutes

Servings: 2

Ingredients:

- 2 tbsp. Olive Oil

- 1 clove of Garlic, peeled & minced

- ½ cup Vegetable Stock

- 1 tsp. Thyme, dried

- 15 oz. Black Beans

- 1 2/3 cup Water, hot

- oz. Mushrooms

- 1 Onion, finely chopped

- 4 Sourdough Bread Slices

- Vegan Butter, to serve

Directions:

1. To begin with, spoon the oil into a medium-sized deep saucepan over a medium heat.
2. Once the oil becomes hot, stir in the onion and garlic.
3. Sauté for 5 minutes or until the onion is translucent.
4. Next, spoon in the mushrooms and thyme. Mix well.
5. Cook for another 5 minutes or until dark brown.
6. Then, pour the water into the mixture along with the stock and beans.
7. Allow it to simmer for 20 minutes or until the mushroom is soft.
8. Pour the mixture to a high-speed blender and pulse for 1 to 2 minutes until it is smooth yet grainy.
9. Serve and enjoy.

Nutrition: Calories: 400 Fat: 32 Fiber: 6 Carbs: 4 Protein: 25

Broccoli Soup

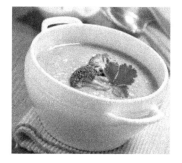

Preparation Time: 5 Minutes

Cooking Time: 15 Minutes

Servings: 2

Ingredients:

- 3 cup Vegetable Broth
- 2 Green Chili
- 2 cups Broccoli Florets
- 1 tbsp. Chia Seeds
- 1 cup Spinach
- 1 tsp. Oil
- 4 Celery Stalk
- 1 Potato, medium & cubed
- 4 Garlic cloves
- Salt, as needed
- Juice of ½ of 1 Lemon

Directions:

1. First, heat the oil in a large sauté pan over a medium-high heat.

2. Once the oil becomes hot, add the potatoes to it.

3. When the potatoes become soft, stir all the remaining ingredients into the pan, excluding the spinach, chia seeds, and lemon.

4. Cook until the broccoli is soft, and then add the spinach and chia seed to the pan.

5. Turn off the heat after cooking for 2 minutes.

6. Allow the spinach mixture to cool slightly. Pour the mixture into a high-speed blender and blend for two minutes or until smooth.

7. Pour the lemon juice over the soup. Stir and serve immediately.

8. Enjoy.

Nutrition: Calories: 200 Fat: 3 Fiber: 2 Carbs: 5 Protein: 4

Mexican Soup

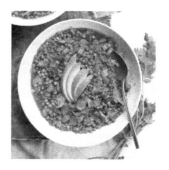

Preparation Time: 10 Minutes

Cooking Time: 45 Minutes

Servings: 6

Ingredients:

- 2 tbsp. Extra Virgin Olive Oil
- 8 oz. can of Diced Tomatoes & Chilies
- 1 Yellow Onion, diced
- 2 cups Green Lentils
- ½ tsp. Salt
- 2 Celery Stalks, diced
- 8 cups Vegetable Broth
- 2 Carrots, peeled & diced
- 2 cups Diced Tomatoes & Juices
- 3 Garlic cloves, minced
- 1 Red Bell Pepper, diced
- 1 tsp. Oregano

- 1 tbsp. Cumin
- ¼ tsp. Smoked Paprika
- 1 Avocado, pitted & diced

Directions:

1. Heat oil in a large-sized pot over a medium heat.
2. Once the oil becomes hot, stir in the onion, bell pepper, carrot, and celery into the pot.
3. Cook the onion mixture for 5 minutes or until the veggies are soft.
4. Then, spoon in garlic, oregano, cumin, and paprika into it and sauté for one minute or until aromatic.
5. Next, add the tomatoes, salt, chilies, broth, and lentils to the mixture.
6. Now, bring the tomato-chili mixture to a boil and allow it to simmer for 32 to 40 minutes or until the lentils become soft.
7. Check the seasoning and add more if needed.
8. Serve along with avocado and hot sauce.

Nutrition: Calories: 344 Fat: 23 Fiber: 12 Carbs: 3 Protein: 16

Celery Dill Soup

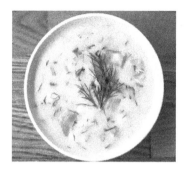

Preparation Time: 10 Minutes

Cooking Time: 20 Minutes

Servings: 4

Ingredients:

- 2 tbsp. coconut oil
- ½ lb. celery root, trimmed
- 1 garlic clove
- 1 medium white onion
- ¼ cup fresh dill, roughly chopped
- 1 tsp cumin powder
- ¼ tsp nutmeg powder
- 1 small head cauliflower, cut into florets
- 3½ cups seasoned vegetable stock
- 5 oz. vegan butter
- Juice from 1 lemon
- ¼ cup coconut cream

- Salt and black pepper to taste

Directions:

1. Melt the coconut oil in a large pot and sauté the celery root, garlic, and onion until softened and fragrant, 5 minutes.

2. Stir in the dill, cumin, and nutmeg, and stir-fry for 1 minute. Mix in the cauliflower and vegetable stock. Allow the soup to boil for 15 minutes and turn the heat off.

3. Add the vegan butter and lemon juice, and puree the soup using an immersion blender.

4. Stir in the coconut cream, salt, black pepper, and dish the soup.

5. Serve warm.

Nutrition: Calories: 180 Fat: 12 Fiber: 4 Carbs: 5 Protein: 17

Medley of Mushroom Soup

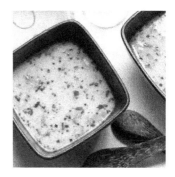

Preparation Time: 10 Minutes

Cooking Time: 20 Minutes

Servings: 4

Ingredients:

- 4 oz. unsalted vegan butter
- 1 small onion, finely chopped
- 1 garlic clove, minced
- 2 cups sliced mixed mushrooms
- ½ lb. celery root, chopped
- ½ tsp dried rosemary
- 3 cups of water
- 1 vegan stock cube, crushed
- 1 tbsp. plain vinegar
- 1 cup coconut cream
- 6 leaves basil, chopped

Directions:

1. Melt the vegan butter in a medium pot and sauté the onion, garlic, mushrooms, celery, and rosemary until the vegetables soften, 5 minutes.

2. Stir in the water, stock cube, and vinegar. Cover the pot, allow boiling, and then, simmer for 10 minutes.

3. Mix in the coconut cream and puree the ingredients using an immersion blender until smooth. Simmer for 2 minutes.

4. Dish the soup and serve warm.

Nutrition: Calories: 140 Fat: 3 Fiber: 2 Carbs: 1. 5 Protein: 7

BREAD RECIPES

Delicious Cheese Bread

Preparation Time: 10 Minutes

Cooking Time: 35 Minutes

Servings: 12

Ingredients:

- Eggs – 2

- All-purpose flour – 2 cups

- Butter – 1/2 cup, melted

- Buttermilk – 1 cup

- Baking soda – 1/2 teaspoon.

- Baking powder – 1/2 teaspoon.

- Sugar – 1 teaspoon.

- Cheddar cheese – 1 cup, shredded

- Salt– 1/2 teaspoon.

Directions:

1. Preheat the oven for 350 F. In a large mixing bowl, mix flour, baking soda, baking powder, sugar, cheese, pepper, and salt.

2. In a small bowl, beat eggs with buttermilk, and butter. Add egg mixture to the flour mixture and mix well.

3. Transfer mixture into the greased 9*5-inch loaf pan and bake in preheated oven for 35-40 minutes.

4. Allow to cool for 15 minutes. Slice and serve.

Nutrition: Calories 202, Carbs 17.6g, Fat 11.9g, Protein 6.2g

Strawberry Bread

Preparation Time: 15 Minutes

Cooking Time: 60 Minutes

Servings: 10

Ingredients:

- Eggs – 2
- All-purpose flour – 2 cups
- Vanilla – 1 teaspoon.
- Vegetable oil – 1/2 cup
- Baking soda – 1 teaspoon.
- Cinnamon – 1/2 teaspoon.
- Brown sugar – 1/2 cup
- White sugar – 1/2 cup
- Fresh strawberries – 2 1/4 cups, chopped
- Salt – 1/2 teaspoon.

Directions:

1. Preheat the oven to 350 F. Grease 9.5-inch loaf pan and set aside.

2. In a mixing bowl, mix together flour, baking soda, cinnamon, brown sugar, white sugar, and salt.

3. In a separate bowl, beat eggs, vanilla, and oil. Stir in strawberries.

4. Add flour mixture to the egg mixture and stir until well combined.

5. Pour batter into the prepared loaf pan and bake in preheated oven for 50-60 minutes.

6. Allow to cool for 10-15 minutes. Slice and serve.

Nutrition: Calories 364, Carbs 40.1g, Fat 21.g, Protein 4.2g

Moist Banana Bread

Preparation Time: 10 Minutes

Cooking Time: 60 Minutes

Servings: 6

Ingredients:

- Eggs – 2
- Baking powder – 1 teaspoon.
- Sugar – 1/2 cup
- Vanilla – 1 teaspoon.
- Butter – 1/2 cup, melted
- Ripe bananas – 3
- All-purpose flour – 1 1/2 cups
- Pinch of salt

Directions:

1. Preheat the oven to 350 F. In a large bowl, add bananas and mash until smooth. Add eggs, vanilla, butter, and mix well.

2. Add flour, baking powder, sugar, and salt and mix until well combined.

3. Pour batter into the greased loaf pan and bake in a preheated oven for 60 minutes. Slice and serve.

Nutrition: Calories 388, Carbs 54.6g, Fat 17.3g, Protein 5.9g

Jalapeno Cheese Bread

Preparation Time: 10 Minutes

Cooking Time: 60 Minutes

Servings: 8

Ingredients:

- Egg – 1
- Flour – 2 cups
- Jalapeno pepper – 1, minced
- Cheddar cheese – 1 1/4 cups, shredded
- Butter – 1/4 cup, melted
- Milk – 1/4 cup
- Yogurt – 3/4 cup
- Sugar – 2 tablespoons.
- Baking soda – 1/2 teaspoon.
- Baking powder– 1 1/2 teaspoon.
- Salt – 1/2 teaspoon.

Directions:

1. Preheat the oven to 350 F. In a bowl, mix together flour, sugar, baking soda, baking powder, and salt.

2. In a separate bowl, whisk together egg, milk, butter, and yogurt. Add egg mixture into the flour mixture and mix until well combined.

3. Stir in jalapeno, and shredded cheese. Pour batter into the parchment-lined 9.5-inch baking tin and bake for 1 hour.

4. Allow to cool for 10-15 minutes. Slice and serve.

Nutrition: Calories 276, Carbs 29.6g, Fat 12.9g, Protein 9.9g

Jalapeno Bread

Preparation Time: 5 Minutes

Cooking Time: 15 Minutes

Servings: 4

Ingredients:

- Eggs – 4
- Jalapeno chilies – 4, chopped
- Baking powder – 1/4 teaspoon.
- Coconut flour – 1/3 cup
- Cheddar cheese – 1/2 cup, grated
- Parmesan cheese – 1/4 cup, grated
- Pepper – 1/2 teaspoon.
- Garlic powder – 1/2 teaspoon.
- Water – 1/4 cup
- Butter – 1/4 cup
- Salt – 1/2 teaspoon.

Directions:

1. Preheat the oven to 400 F. In a bowl, whisk together eggs, pepper, salt, water, and butter.
2. Add baking powder, garlic powder, and coconut flour and mix until well combined. Add jalapenos, cheddar cheese, and parmesan cheese.

3. Mix well and season with pepper. Line baking tray with parchment pepper. Pour batter into a baking tray and bake for 15 minutes.

4. Slice and serve.

Nutrition: Calories 250, Carbs 3g, Fat 22g, Protein 11g

Banana Zucchini Bread

Preparation Time: 10 Minutes

Cooking Time: 45 Minutes

Servings: 12

Ingredients:

- Eggs – 4

- Cinnamon – 1 tablespoon.

- Baking soda – 3/4 teaspoon.

- Coconut flour – 1/2 cup

- Coconut oil – 1 tablespoon.

- Banana – 1, mashed

- Stevia – 1 teaspoon.

- Zucchini – 1 cup, shredded and squeezed out all liquid

- Walnuts – 1/2 cup, chopped

- Apple cider vinegar – 1 teaspoon.

- Nutmeg – 1/2 teaspoon.

- Salt – 1/2 teaspoon.

Directions:

1. Preheat the oven to 350 F. Grease loaf pan with oil and set aside. In a large bowl, whisk together egg, banana, oil, and stevia.

2. Add all dry Ingredients, vinegar, and zucchini and stir until smooth. Add walnuts and stir well. Pour batter into the loaf pan and bake for 45 minutes.

3. Slice and serve.

Nutrition: Calories 78, Carbs 4.4g, Fat 5.8g, Protein 3.4g

Broccoli Bread

Preparation Time: 10 Minutes

Cooking Time: 30 Minutes

Servings: 5

Ingredients:

- Eggs – 5, lightly beaten
- Broccoli florets – 3/4 cup, chopped
- Cheddar cheese – 1 cup, shredded
- Baking powder – 2 teaspoons.
- Coconut flour – 3 1/1 tablespoons.
- Salt – 1 teaspoon.

Directions:

1. Preheat the oven to 350 F. Grease loaf pan with butter and set aside. Add all Ingredients into the bowl and mix well.
2. Pour egg mixture into the prepared loaf pan and bake for 30 minutes.
3. Slice and serve.

Nutrition: Calories 205, Carbs 8g, Fat 13g, Protein 13g

Almond Bread

Preparation Time: 10 Minutes

Cooking Time: 30 Minutes

Servings: 20

Ingredients:

- Eggs – 6, separated
- Cream of tartar – 1/4 teaspoon.
- Baking powder – 3 teaspoon.
- Butter – 4 tablespoons, melted
- Almond flour – 1 1/2 cups
- Salt – 1/4 teaspoon.

Directions:

1. Preheat the oven to 375 F. Grease 8*4-inch loaf pan with butter and set aside. Add egg whites and cream of tartar in a large bowl and beat until soft peaks form.

2. Add almond flour, baking powder, egg yolks, butter, and salt in a food processor and process until combined.

3. Add 1/3 of egg white mixture into the almond flour mixture and process until combined. Now add remaining egg white mixture and process gently to combine.

4. Pour batter into the prepared loaf pan and bake for 30 minutes. Slice and serve.

Nutrition: Calories 52, Carbs 1g, Fat 4g, Protein 2g

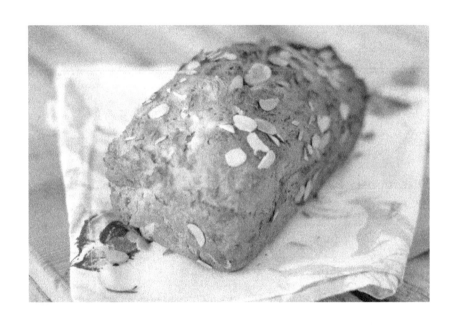

Sandwich Bread

Preparation Time: 20 Minutes

Cooking Time: 50 Minutes

Servings: 12

Ingredients:

- Coconut flour – 1/2 cup
- Apple cider vinegar – 1 teaspoon.
- Water – 3/4 cup
- Olive oil – 4 tablespoons.
- Eggs – 5
- Baking soda – 1 teaspoon
- Almond flour – 2 cups + 2 tablespoons.
- Salt – 1/2 teaspoon

Directions:

1. Preheat the oven to 350 F. Grease loaf pan and set aside. In a large bowl, combine together almond flour, baking soda, coconut flour, and salt. Set aside.

2. Beat eggs in another bowl until frothy. Add vinegar, water, and oil in egg mixture and process until well combined.

3. Add all dry **Ingredients:** and process until smooth. Pour batter into the prepared loaf pan and bake for 50 minutes. Slice and serve.

Nutrition: Calories 125, Carbs 2.5g, Fat 11.5g, Protein 4.7g

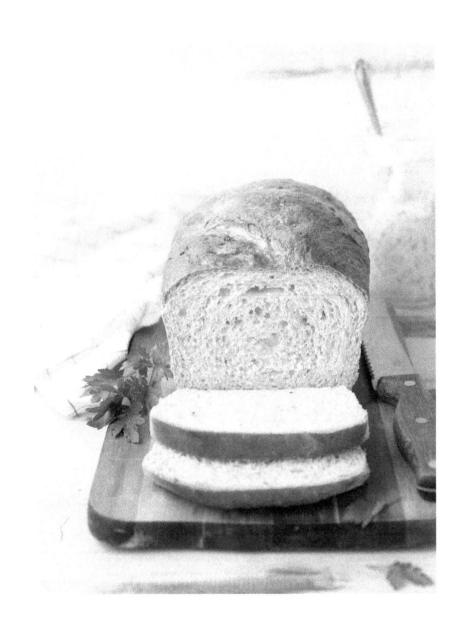

Sweet Rolls

Preparation Time: 2 hours

Cooking Time: 30 Minutes

Servings: 8

Ingredients:

- 2 tablespoons cane sugar
- 1 teaspoon rapid dry yeast
- 2 1/2 tablespoons warm water
- 1/2 cup pineapple juice, plus more for brushing tops of rolls
- 2 tablespoons coconut oil, melted
- 1 3/4 cups unbleached all-purpose flour, plus more for rolling out the dough

Directions:

1. In a small bowl, combine the sugar, yeast, and warm water. Stir gently and set aside for 10 minutes.
2. In another small bowl, combine 1/2 cup of pineapple juice and the coconut oil and stir.
3. Add the yeast mixture to the pineapple mixture and stir gently.
4. Add 1 3/4 cups of flour, and mix with your hands until well combined. The dough should not be too sticky. Knead in the bowl for 10 minutes, or until the dough is soft and smooth.
5. Place the dough in an oiled bowl, cover with a clean, damp towel, and place in a warm area for 1 hour to allow it to rise.

6. On a lightly floured surface, knead the dough, incorporating the flour from the surface. Break the dough into 8 equal pieces and form rolls.

7. Place the rolls on an oiled baking pan and allow to rise again for 30 to 40 minutes. Twenty minutes into this second rise, preheat the oven to 375 degree F.

8. Use a pastry brush to brush the tops of the rolls with pineapple juice.

9. Bake for 25 to 30 minutes or until golden brown.

Nutrition: Calories 115, Carbs 2.5g, Fat 11.5g, Protein 6.7g

Cornbread Waffles

Preparation Time: 6 Minutes

Cooking Time: 10 Minutes

Servings: 5

Ingredients:

- 1/3cup unsweetened plant-based milk
- 1 teaspoon apple cider vinegar
- 1/2 teaspoon baking powder
- 1/2 teaspoon baking soda
- 1 cup fine cornmeal
- 1/2 cup masa
- 1 cup unbleached all-purpose flour
- 1/3 cup unsweetened applesauce
- 1/4 cup sunflower oil
- Coconut oil cooking spray

Directions:

1. In a small bowl, whisk together the milk and vinegar and set aside.

2. In another small bowl, whisk the baking powder, baking soda, cornmeal, masa, and flour together.

3. Add the applesauce and oil to the bowl containing the milk and stir to mix.

4. Pour the wet Ingredients into the dry Ingredients and whisk until well combined.

5. Turn a waffle iron on and coat with cooking spray.

6. When the iron is hot, pour in enough batter to fill the waffle iron and cook for 4 to 5 minutes, or until lightly golden brown.

7. Take the waffle out of the waffle iron and cut it in half. Repeat with the remaining batter

Nutrition: Calories 175, Carbs 2.5g, Fat 9.5g, Protein 5.7g

Buttermilk Biscuits

Preparation Time: 15 Minutes

Cooking Time: 15 Minutes

Servings: 8

Ingredients:

- 1 cup plant-based milk
- 1 tablespoon apple cider vinegar
- 2 cups unbleached all-purpose flour, plus more for cutting out the biscuits
- 1 tablespoon baking powder
- 1/2 teaspoon baking soda
- 1/2 teaspoon salt
- 1 tablespoon cane sugar
- 4 tablespoons (1/2 stick) Earth Balance vegan butter, cold

Directions:

1. Preheat the oven to 450 degree F and line a baking pan with parchment paper.
2. In a small bowl, mix the milk and vinegar and allow to curdle, usually no more than 5 minutes.
3. In a medium mixing bowl, whisk together the flour, baking powder, baking soda, salt, and sugar.

4. Add the cold butter and use your fingers or a pastry cutter to combine until only small pieces remain and the mixture looks grainy, like sand. Work fast so the butter doesn't get too soft.

5. Make a well in the dry Ingredients, and use a wooden spoon to stir gently while pouring in the milk mixture 1/4 cup at a time. Stir until well combined.

6. Sprinkle flour on a clean surface and dump the dough onto it. Dust the top of the dough with flour. Gently flatten the dough with your hands until it is about 1 inch thick, then dip a coffee mug rim into the flour to coat it and use it to cut out the biscuits.

7. Place the cut biscuits on the lined baking pan, and bake for 6 minutes, then turn and bake another 6 minutes or until the tops and edges turn golden brown.

Nutrition: Calories 115, Carbs 2.5g, Fat 10.5g, Protein 4.7g

Banana-Lemon Loaf

Preparation Time: 15 minutes

Cooking Time: 1.5 hours

Serving Size: 1 ounce (28.3g)

Ingredients:

- 2 cups all-purpose flour
- 1 cup bananas, very ripe and mashed
- 1 cup walnuts, chopped
- 1 cup of sugar
- One tablespoon baking powder
- One teaspoon lemon peel, grated
- ½ teaspoon salt
- Two eggs
- ½ cup of vegetable oil
- Two tablespoons lemon juice

Direction:

1. Put all ingredients into a pan in this order: bananas, wet ingredients, and then dry ingredients.
2. Press the "Quick" or "Cake" setting of your bread machine.
3. Allow the cycles to be completed.

4. Take out the pan from the machine. The cooldown for 10
   minutes before slicing the bread enjoy.

Nutrition: Calories: 120 | Carbohydrates: 15g Fat: 6g | Protein:
2g

Orange Date Bread

Preparation Time: 20 minutes

Cooking Time: 1.5 hours

Serving Size: 1 ounce (28.3g)

Ingredients:

- 2 cups all-purpose flour
- 1 cup dates, chopped
- ¾ cup of sugar
- ½ cup walnuts, chopped
- Two tablespoons orange rind, grated
- 1 ½ teaspoons baking powder
- One teaspoon baking soda
- ½ cup of orange juice
- ½ cup of water
- One tablespoon vegetable oil
- One teaspoon vanilla extract

Direction:

1. Put the wet ingredients then the dry ingredients into the bread pan.
2. Press the "Quick" or "Cake" mode of the bread machine.
3. Allow all cycles to be finished.

4. Remove the pan from the machine, but keep the bread in the pan for 10 minutes more.

5. Take out the bread from the pan, and let it cool down completely before slicing.

Nutrition: Calories: 80 | Carbohydrates: 14g Fat: 2g | Protein: 1g

Zero-Fat Carrot Pineapple Loaf

Preparation Time: 20 minutes

Cooking Time: 1.5 hours

Serving Size: 1 ounce (28.3g)

Ingredients:

- 2 ½ cups all-purpose flour
- ¾ cup of sugar
- ½ cup pineapples, crushed
- ½ cup carrots, grated
- ½ cup raisins
- Two teaspoons baking powder
- ½ teaspoon ground cinnamon
- ½ teaspoon salt
- ¼ teaspoon allspice
- ¼ teaspoon nutmeg
- ½ cup applesauce
- One tablespoon molasses

Direction:

1. Put first the wet ingredients into the bread pan before the dry ingredients.

2. Press the "Quick" or "Cake" mode of your bread machine.

3. Allow the machine to complete all cycles.

4. Take out the pan from the machine, but wait for another 10 minutes before transferring the bread into a wire rack.

5. Cooldown the bread before slicing.

Nutrition: Calories: 70 | Carbohydrates: 16g Fat: 0g | Protein: 1g

Autumn Treasures Loaf

Preparation Time: 15 minutes

Cooking Time: 1/5 hours

Serving Size: 1 ounce (28.3g)

Ingredients:

- 1 cup all-purpose flour
- ½ cup dried fruit, chopped
- ¼ cup pecans, chopped
- ¼ cup of sugar
- Two tablespoons baking powder
- One teaspoon salt
- ¼ teaspoon of baking soda
- ½ teaspoon ground nutmeg
- 1 cup apple juice
- ¼ cup of vegetable oil
- Three tablespoons aquafaba
- One teaspoon of vanilla extract

Direction:

1. Add all wet ingredients first to the bread pan before the dry ingredients.

2. Turn on the bread machine with the "Quick" or "Cake" setting.

3. Wait for all cycles to be finished.

4. Remove the bread pan from the machine.

5. After 10 minutes, transfer the bread from the pan into a wire rack.

6. Slice the bread only when it has completely cooled down.

Nutrition: Calories: 80 | Carbohydrates: 12g Fat: 3g | Protein: 1g

Conclusion

Vegan recipes do not need to be boring. There are so many different combinations of veggies, fruits, whole grains, beans, seeds, and nuts that you will be able to make unique meal plans for many months. These recipes contain the instructions along with the necessary ingredients and nutritional information.

If you ever come across someone complaining that they can't follow the plant-based diet because it's expensive, hard to cater for, lacking in variety, or tasteless, feel free to have them take a look at this book. In no time, you'll have another companion walking beside you on this road to healthier eating and better living.

Although healthy, many people are still hesitant to give vegan food a try. They mistakenly believe that these would be boring, tasteless, and complicated to make. This is the farthest thing from the truth.

Fruits and vegetables are organically delicious, fragrant, and vibrantly colored. If you add herbs, mushrooms, and nuts to the mix, dishes will always come out packed full of flavor it only takes a bit of effort and time to prepare great-tasting vegan meals for your family.

How easy was that? Don't we all want a seamless and easy way to cook like this?

I believe cooking is taking a better turn and the days, when we needed so many ingredients to provide a decent meal, were gone. Now, with easy tweaks, we can make delicious, quick, and easy meals. Most importantly, we get to save a bunch of cash on groceries.

I am grateful for downloading this book and taking the time to read it. I know that you have learned a lot and you had a great time reading it. Writing books is the best way to share the skills I have with your and the best tips too.

I know that there are many books and choosing my book is amazing. I am thankful that you stopped and took time to decide. You made a great decision and I am sure that you enjoyed it.

I will be even happier if you will add some comments. Feedbacks helped by growing and they still do. They help me to choose better content and new Ideas. So, maybe your feedback can trigger an idea for my next book.

Hopefully, this book has helped you understand that vegetarian recipes and diet can improve your life, not only by improving your health and helping you lose weight, but also by saving you money and time. I sincerely hope that the recipes provided in this book have proven to be quick, easy, and delicious, and have provided you with enough variety to keep your taste buds interested and curious.

I hope you enjoyed reading about my book!

CPSIA information can be obtained
at www.ICGtesting.com
Printed in the USA
BVHW041952230421
605736BV00015B/520